MULTIPLE BIRTHS

MULTIPLE BIRTHS

BY ELAINE LANDAU

A First Book

FRANKLIN WATTS   A Division of Grolier Publishing
New York / London / Hong Kong / Sydney / Danbury, Connecticut

FOR MICHAEL

Interior and cover design: Michelle Regan
Cover illustration: Victoria Vebell
Photographs ©: Ben Klaffke: 21, 22 bottom, 23, 43, 48, 49, 51; Diamond Institute: 38 (Hollander Photographic Services), 26 top, 33; Photo Researchers: 22 top (Mark C. Burnett), 40 (Nicholas Desciose), 29 (Spencer Grant), 27 (James King-Holmes/SPL), 26 bottom (Hank Morgan), 36 (Peter Ryan/SPL); UPI/Corbis-Bettmann: 8, 9, 11, 13, 15, 17, 18; Woodfin Camp & Associates: 32 (Paula Lerner).

**Visit Franklin Watts on the Internet at:
http://publishing.grolier.com**

Library of Congress Cataloging-in-Publication Data

Landau, Elaine.
Multiple births / by Elaine Landau.
p.   cm. — (A First book)
Includes bibliographical references and index.
Summary: Explores the phenomenon of multiple births, including those of twins, triplets, and larger groupings, discussing possible causes, medical issues, effects on the families, and other moral and practical concerns.
ISBN 0-531-20309-3
1. Multiple birth—Juvenile literature. [1. Multiple birth.] I. Title. II. Series.
RG696.L36   1997
618.2'5—dc21

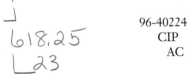

96-40224
CIP
AC

CONTENTS

CHAPTER 1

THE TOAST OF CANADA

*W*hen Elzire Dionne, the 25-year-old wife of a struggling French-Canadian farmer, learned she was pregnant, she was surprised, but not shaken by the news. She had given birth before—this would be her sixth child. And she knew that somehow she would make room for the baby in her family's cramped, unheated farmhouse.

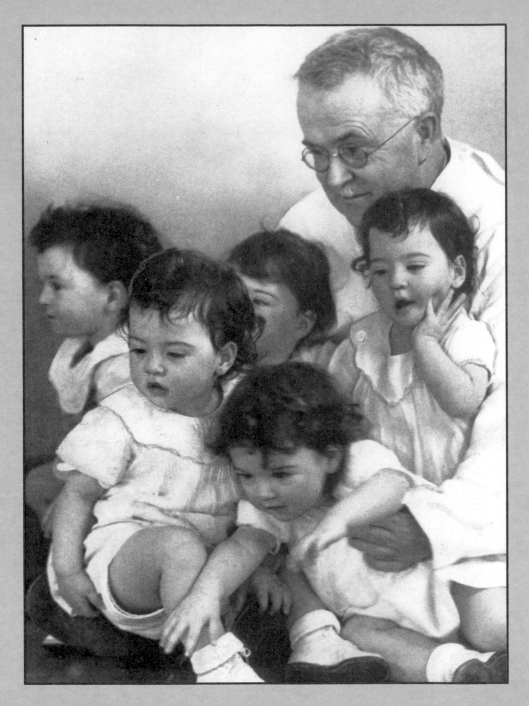

Dr. Allan Dafoe embraces the five Dionne quintuplets on their first birthday.

But Elzire did not have an easy pregnancy. Although the baby wasn't due until July, Elzire had already become extremely large by early May. Her legs had swollen to nearly twice their normal size. She had been warned by Dr. Allan Roy Dafoe, the local doctor, to stay off her feet and get plenty of rest. But this was difficult for Elzire. It was 1934, times were tough economically, and the Dionnes could not afford household help.

In any case, before long, things changed. Early one May morning, nearly two months before Elzire was due to give birth, she went into labor. Thinking this birth would be routine, only the usual two **midwives** came to assist with the delivery. As it turned out, there was nothing ordinary about this seemingly everyday event. Elzire Dionne did not give birth to a single child, twins, or even triplets. Instead, she had five identical baby girls—even though the odds of doing so at the time were 44 million to 1.

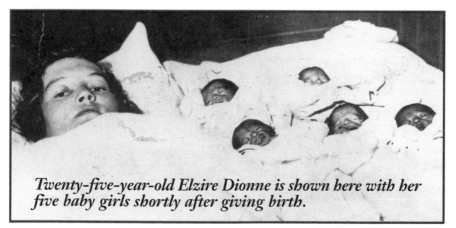

Twenty-five-year-old Elzire Dionne is shown here with her five baby girls shortly after giving birth.

Five Tiny Infants

After the first two infants were born, Dr. Dafoe arrived to deliver the remaining three. Because they were born **prematurely**, all five girls were extremely tiny, and their survival was doubtful. A midwife rubbed warm olive oil on the infants, wrapped them in blankets, and placed them snugly in a basket set directly in front of a warm oven.

Dafoe thought the babies might die before morning, but he was wrong. Even though each was practically small enough to fit in an adult's palm, the Dionne quintuplets survived and thrived. And as word of the miraculous birth leaked to the public and press, their lives and those of their family members would never be the same.

Actually, word of the girls' arrival spread innocently enough. A relative of the Dionnes had called a newspaper to learn whether a birth announcement for five babies would cost more than one for a single birth. After the newspaper called Dr. Dafoe to confirm the incredible account, the media wheels sprang into action.

Today we are used to hearing about multiple births, but in the 1930s, the Dionne quintuplets were headline material. Reporters from near and far headed for the Canadian backwoods farmhouse, and before long, hoards of people followed.

On the advice of Dafoe and the local parish priest, Oliva Dionne, the quintuplets' father, agreed to let a show-business promoter put the girls on exhibit. In return

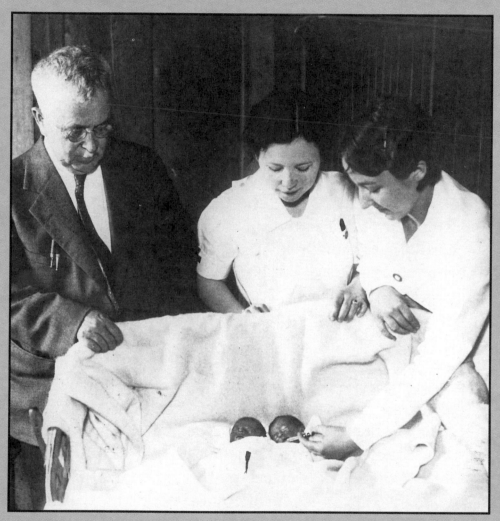

Two nurses feed the babies with an eyedropper as Dr. Dafoe looks on.

for allowing the infants to be publicly displayed, Dionne was to receive 23 cents of the price of each admission ticket.

The Government Steps In

But the French-Canadian farmer and father of ten never collected these fees. The public outcry against such "blatant **profiteering**" was so widespread that the Canadian government stepped in. Further claiming that the unsanitary conditions of the farmhouse could be dangerous to the infants' health, the authorities took the girls away from their family and made them wards of the state. A board of guardians appointed to safeguard their welfare included Dr. Dafoe, but not the infants' parents. Suddenly the Dionnes no longer had any say in how the "quints," as the children came to be called, would be brought up.

As one Canadian author wrote, "Their [the quints'] parents were viewed as nothing more than a nuisance, a pair of barely competent French-Canadian rustics."[1] However, the government's presence in the girls' lives would hardly prove to be beneficial for them. And while Oliva Dionne had been scorned for wishing to exhibit the infants, the government eventually did just that.

The authorities removed the quints to a building that had been constructed on Oliva Dionne's property just across the road from the family farmhouse. Yet this did not bring the girls closer to their parents. The Dionnes were frequently told not to kiss the quintuplets or even touch them for fear of exposing the girls to germs.

"Quintland"

As time passed, this nine-room structure was expanded into a full-fledged tourist facility known as Quintland. Streams of tourists filed by the glass observation area daily to sneak a peek at the young girls at play.

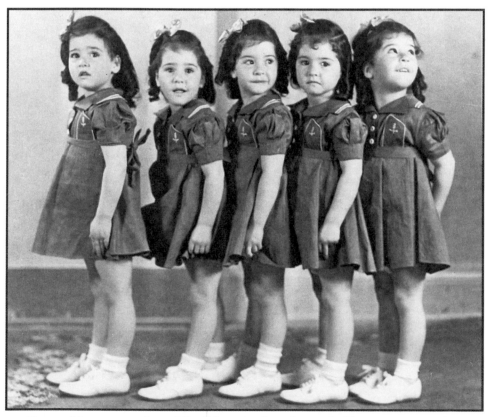

Dressed in cute outfits with ribbons in their hair, the Dionne quintuplets became a highly valued tourist draw.

Undeniably, the Dionne quintuplets were a major tourist draw. Each day, thousands of visitors paid to see them, providing a much-needed boost to the sagging local economy. To accommodate the crowds, crews were hired to construct and pave local routes as well as install new power lines. The quints' popularity and drawing power also brought a host of new jobs and business opportunities to the region.

Food stands and souvenir stands sprang up rapidly along with an assortment of other shops and services geared to the travelers' needs. Many of those who had seen the quints up close or knew the quints' family eagerly accepted money for newspaper interviews. For a price, one of the midwives who helped deliver the quints displayed the basket she had placed the infants in shortly after their birth. "We all had a new life because of the quints," one neighbor noted in describing the end result of the children's birth.[2]

In time, the Dionne quintuplets became the largest tourist attraction in North America—claiming more visitors than the famous honeymoon haven, Niagara Falls.[3] Images of the adorable curly-haired, dimpled darlings could be seen almost everywhere. They made the covers of such widely circulated magazines as *Time* and *Life*. They appeared in films and on the radio. There were even Dionne quintuplets dolls for sale. The Canadian government allowed the girls to be used in **endorsements** for a broad range of products.

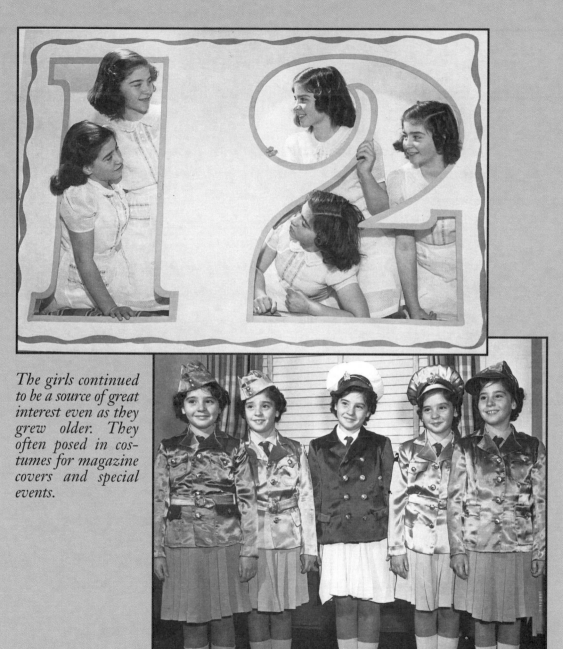

The girls continued to be a source of great interest even as they grew older. They often posed in costumes for magazine covers and special events.

The quints were big moneymakers, but unfortunately, they did not keep much of what they earned. While the public believed that the government paid for Quintland and other related expenses, this wasn't so. A relative of the quintuplets described the actual situation this way: "Their guardians took their fees out of the money [earned by the girls]. They [the quints] paid for the salaries of the staff at Quintland and all of the costs of the day-to-day operations of the place. It cost them $200,000 to build that ridiculous observatory. They [the girls] were even charged $5,000 for the construction of a toilet for the public."[4]

Back at Home
The family was finally reunited in 1943, after a three-story yellow-brick home was built for all of them on the Dionne farm. By then, Elzire and Oliva had had more children, bringing the total number of Dionne youngsters to 13. Although everyone eagerly looked forward to being a "normal" family, relationships between family members became strained. Some of the quints' brothers and sisters bitterly resented the anguish their parents had been put through by the government's accusations. As one of the quints' sisters said, "They [Oliva and Elzire Dionne] cried day after day. My youth ended because there was so much suffering."[5]

The difference between how the quintuplets and their

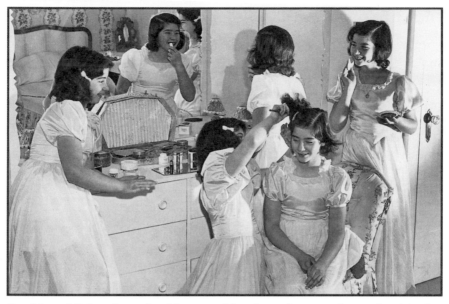

In this publicity shot, the 12-year-old quintuplets are shown having fun playing "dress up" with their mother's makeup kit.

siblings had been brought up served to further deepen the family rift. Learning early on that they would have to work hard to ensure their survival and future, the other Dionne children had always helped with farm chores, cooking, cleaning, laundry, and child care. The quints, on the other hand, had become used to being indulged and adored. According to Cécile, one of the Dionne quintuplets, "When we were very young we were treated iike princesses. We didn't know it at the time, but we didn't care either. We were happy."[6]

However, she notes that their lives took a turn for the worse once they were reunited with a family in which they no longer fit. "It was not an easy situation," she remembered. "We lived separate lives. But there was always so much tension in our relationships, always so many quarrels. Our brothers and sisters, even our parents, always clung to the idea that we were the cause of their misery and unhappiness."[7] Unfortunately, even today, as older adults, the surviving quintuplets do not enjoy a warm relationship with their other siblings.

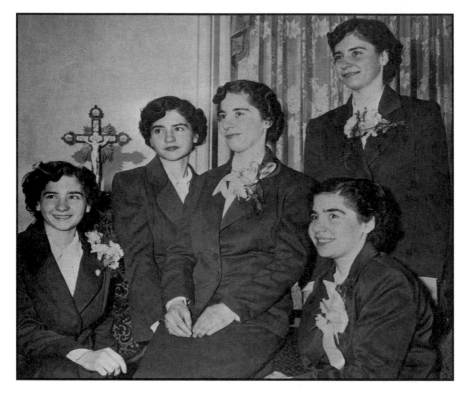

Still wearing identical outfits, the Dionne quintuplets pose for a picture as young women.

The Quints as Adults

As the quintuplets matured, the question of money also became a sensitive issue. During their youth, the government set up a trust for the quints that was to be made available to them when they turned 21. Although $1 million dollars was supposedly placed in the account, only $800,000 was left by the time the quints were ready to receive the money. No one is sure what happened to the rest. Some say that the girls lost interest payments on some long-term investments and that the fund established for their future lacked an inflation clause. The girls' father has also been blamed for squandering the money—a charge that the quints' brothers and sisters firmly deny.

In any case, the surviving quints claim to have suffered a great deal as a result of being deprived of a normal childhood and family life. Only four of the five quints lived to adulthood. Another died at just 36 years of age of a blood clot in her brain. She had become extremely depressed after her marriage ended, and her condition was worsened by excessive drinking. Although crowds had clamored to get a glimpse of her in her youth, she died alone in her apartment. The marriages of two of the other quints ended in divorce as well. As the daughter of one of the midwives who delivered the quints remarked, "The girls grew up in captivity. If only the government had not shown up. The whole family would be happy today."[8]

CHAPTER 2

MORE MULTIPLES

*I*n recent times, few parents of multiples have allowed their children to be taken advantage of as the Dionne sisters were. Today, families with multiples tend to be more aware of the rights and needs of their children. And with multiple births becoming more common, they no longer cause the same level of excitement as in the past.

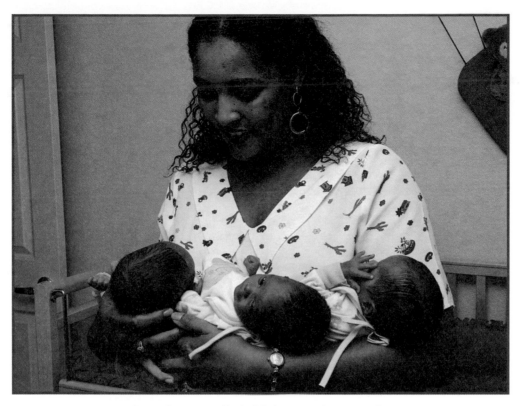

A mother proudly holds her newborn triplets.

Identical and Fraternal Multiples

Just as there are two kinds of twins, there are two types of multiples. Identical multiples occur when a pregnant woman's fertilized **egg** splits into several parts. These develop into separate fetuses with the same genetic makeup. When the children are born, they look just like one another. The Dionne sisters were identical multiples.

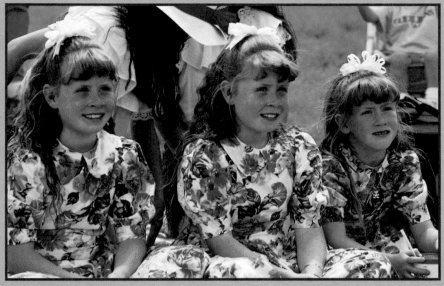

These three "look-alike" sisters are identical multiples.

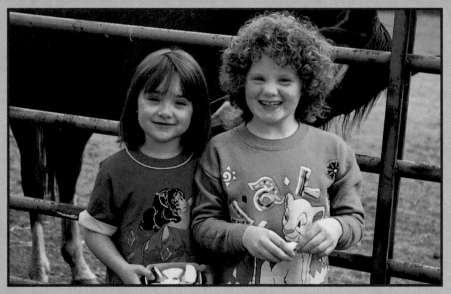

Fraternal multiples, like the fraternal twins seen here, do not necessarily look very much like one another.

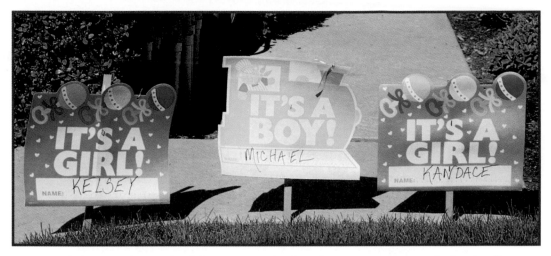

A family places colorful signs outside their home announcing the birth of triplets. Multiples have become increasingly common in recent years.

Much more common are fraternal multiples. These occur when two or more eggs are released by a woman at about the same time and each egg is fertilized by a separate sperm. Although these children will be born on the same day, they will not be any more like each other genetically than other brothers and sisters. These multiples may be all boys or all girls, or a mix of both.

The rise in multiple births has been considerable. At the close of the 1970s, a little more than 68,000 babies were born as twins, triplets, quadruplets, or in larger groupings. A decade later, the number was over 81,000— a whopping 19 percent increase. The numbers have continued to rise and are expected to do so in the 21st century as well. The various reasons for this increase are described in the following pages.

Delaying Pregnancy

Many women now feel it is important to have both a career and a family. This has resulted in large numbers of females delaying pregnancy until they've established themselves in their careers. Women who once might have started having children in their early twenties now often wait until their middle or late thirties or even forties. At the close of the 1980s, women between the ages of 35 and 39 accounted for over 25 percent of all those giving birth.

For some still-unknown reason, women who give birth in their thirties are considerably more likely to have multiples than those who give birth earlier. The odds of having either twins or triplets become highest for women between 35 and 39 years of age.

Commenting on these numbers, Dr. Russell Larson, vice-chairman of Obstetrics, Gynecology, and Reproductive Sciences at the University of California, San Francisco, noted, "As long as women continue to put off having babies until their thirties, we'll see more multiple births."[1]

Using the "Pill" for Birth Control

Women who have taken "the pill" (oral contraceptives) for six months or longer are increasingly likely to have multiples if they become pregnant shortly after discontinuing its use. Studies have shown that these women may nearly double their chances of having multiples. Doctors are not entirely sure why this occurs. However, it's suspected that women experience a strong **hormonal** surge after going off the pill that causes their **ovaries** to release a number of eggs. A pregnancy results when sperm from a male unites with a female's egg during sexual intercourse. If more than one of these eggs is fertilized by the male's sperm, more than one child is conceived. With additional eggs being released, this is increasingly likely to occur.

Infertility Treatments

There's also a connection between the use of fertility drugs and multiple births. Between 1968 and 1982, the number of people seeking help for **infertility** tripled. Many of those seeking such help eventually use fertility drugs. Some fertility drugs stimulate the woman's ovaries to produce additional eggs.

As was discussed above, if more than one egg unites with the male's sperm, multiple births result. The fertility drug Clomid is among those medications most commonly used by women who are having trouble becoming pregnant. Prescriptions for Clomid nearly doubled between 1971 and 1991. An even stronger fertility drug, Pergonal, causes multiple births in 10 to 20 percent of women. In addition, medical studies indicate that the use of other fertility drugs is on the rise.[2]

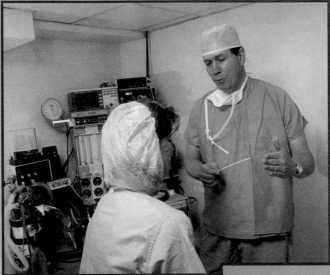

Here a doctor explains to a patient the steps involved in fertility treatments. Some types of infertility treatments are more likely to result in multiples than others.

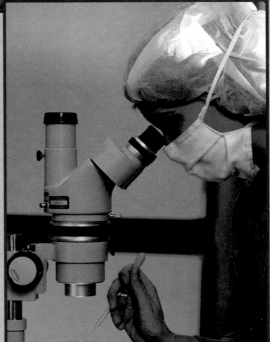

The lab technician shown here monitors the fertilization process in in vitro fertilization.

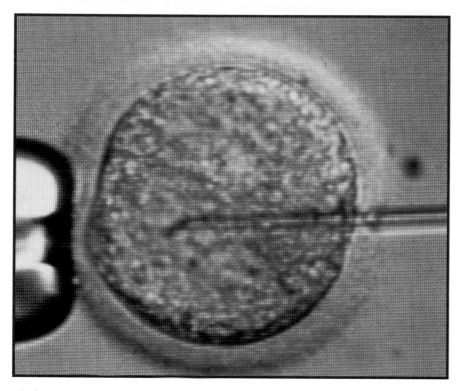

A close-up view of the in vitro fertilization process

Fertility treatments resulting in a high number of multiples was especially evident on November 19, 1997, when Bobbi McCaughey of Iowa became the first woman in known human history to deliver septuplets (seven babies) that lived. Mrs. McCaughey had taken a fertility drug.

Other infertility treatments can have a similar outcome. In the procedure known as **in vitro fertilization (IVF)**, the woman may be given fertility drugs to produce more eggs and hopefully increase the likelihood of one egg fertilizing and developing into a baby. Then a doctor removes these eggs from her ovaries and fertilizes them with the male's sperm in a lab before placing the fertilized eggs back into her body. Several fertilized eggs are transferred in the hope that the procedure will work in at least one instance and a pregnancy will be achieved. But sometimes IVF works too well. More than one of these fertilized eggs implant in the uterus, and multiple births result. As one doctor said about IVF, "We've seen a much higher incidence of triplets as well as twins. The miracle baby can become one of a brood."

Better Health and Medical Care

Improved health, as well as medical advances over the years, have also been factors in the rise in multiple births. A mother's good health can be crucial to the survival and growth of the **fetus** in her womb. Surveys reveal that the majority of women who successfully carry multiples to term tend to be tall and well nourished.

Advances in pregnancy detection have contributed to the increase in multiple births as well. If a woman and her doctor know that there is more than one fetus, they can try to avoid the medical problems that sometimes occur in these situations. The overall result is that a larger number of healthy multiples are born. In the past, multiples were more likely to be **miscarried** or to die at birth.

All these factors have combined to create a change in

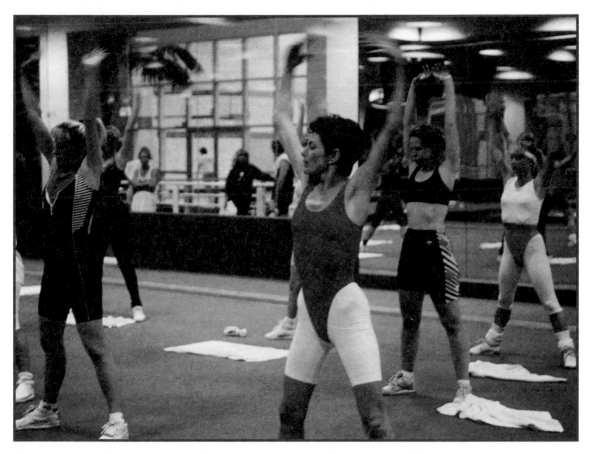

Proper diet and exercise can influence a woman's ability to successfully carry multiples to term.

what happens in hospital delivery rooms each year. Between the early 1970s and 1990, births of triplets in the United States rose by 221 percent. There has been a 65 percent increase in the number of twins born over the last twenty years. Not only are multiple births no longer rare, they may be on their way to becoming commonplace.

CHAPTER 3

TOUGH CHOICES

*F*or couples who have long tried to have a family, news that quadruplets, triplets, or twins are on the way can be an unexpected joy. That's how it was for Denise and Kirk Aymond, who had gone for infertility treatments when they weren't able to have a child on their own. The fertility drugs Denise took were successful, and she was told that she was having quadruplets.

After digesting the news, the couple was actually quite pleased with the idea of a multiple birth. "Everyone said we would be fine with quads," Ms. Aymond recalled. "And fertility treatment is so emotional and so expensive that deep down, you hope for more than one baby."[1]

But before long, their happiness was somewhat tempered. The couple learned that there had been an error in the number of babies predicted. Instead of four fetuses, five had now been detected. The Aymonds were aware of the risks involved. Their physician had explained that in a multiple pregnancy, each additional child heightens the likelihood that all or some of the children won't survive or will have one or more handicaps. Multiple-birth babies are six times as likely to have **cerebral palsy**, and twice as likely to have such birth defects as blindness and brain damage. Even so, the couple looked bravely ahead to the future and hoped for the best.

A Rough Pregnancy

The Aymonds worked closely with the doctors and staff at Women's Hospital in Baton Rouge, Louisiana, to best ensure Denise's health and that of the unborn babies. Yet despite the care she received, Denise still cited her pregnancy as the hardest part of the experience. To reduce the possibility of the babies being born prematurely, she had to leave her job as a registered nurse. Most of her time was spent at home, lying down. As her pregnancy

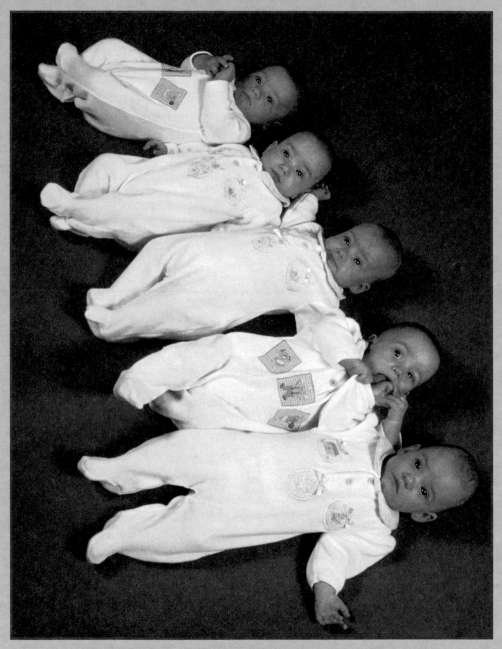

For some couples who have long dreamed of becoming parents, an immediately large family can be a dream come true.

progressed, she was put on 24-hour-a-day bed rest. Within about a three-month period, her weight rose from 145 to 223 pounds (66 to 101 kg). Describing what it was like to carry five infants, she said, "I was miserable, I couldn't move. I felt like a turtle on its back."[2]

Denise's doctors decided to deliver the babies by **cesarean section** about nine weeks prior to their due date. At that point, the doctors felt that Denise's health was at risk. She had developed high blood pressure, and her body was **retaining** fluid.

The doctors, nurses, and other medical personnel who'd prepared for the quints' birth were called to the hospital. Four doctors looked after Ms. Aymond, while each of the babies was assigned a **respiratory therapist** and two **intensive-care** nurses.

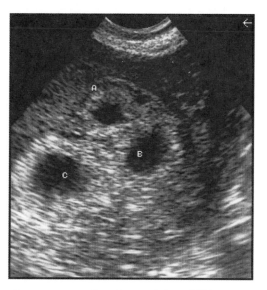

A sonogram showing triplets. This was how the Aymonds learned they were having multiples.

The Need for Special Care

The babies were delivered quickly and rushed to the hospital's intensive-care nursery. Since each of the children weighed more than 2 pounds (0.9 kg), at birth, the doctors felt their chances for survival were good. Yet it was over two months before any of the babies could come home. During that time, each of the quintuplets survived some serious medical problems, including intestinal and blood infections.

The infants' medical emergencies did not stop once they were brought home. The eyesight of one of the quints began to fail before she was three months old. Two other quints had to have strips of bone that had fused too early in their development removed from their skulls.

The Aymonds' medical bills were extremely high. Skyrocketing hospital costs are not uncommon with multiple births. That's because these babies are frequently born prematurely—despite measures to prevent this. Unfortunately, the end result is often small, sick newborns needing huge amounts of costly care.

When a couple from Peoria, Illinois, had premature quintuplets, medical bills reached $2.75 million. Because the babies were born 12 weeks early, their lungs were still very underdeveloped. The infants improved, but three of them had to undergo heart surgery. Still another nearly died battling a serious virus. As is frequently the case, the quints continued to have health problems after coming home from the hospital. One baby had to have her oxygen intake monitored, and another was found to have a mild form of cerebral palsy.

A 1994 study published in the *New England Journal of Medicine* examined the delivery costs for 13,206 women who gave birth at Boston's Brigham and Women's Hospital from 1986 to 1991. The average hospital stay with the birth of a single child was 4.6 days, while mothers of twins were generally hospitalized for about 8.2 days. With three or four or more babies, the mothers' hospital stays tend to be even longer.

The babies' hospital stays were usually longer as well. While only 15 percent of singly born infants needed intensive care, nearly 50 percent of all twins and about 75 percent of the triplets, quadruplets, and quintuplets spent some time in the intensive-care unit.

The effect on the costs involved was inescapable. The Boston study demonstrated that while the hospital costs for a single newborn baby were about $9,850, the average cost for twins was $37,950 ($18,975 per baby). For triplets, the average cost was $109,765 ($36,588 per baby). The researchers estimated that if each of the multiple births in the study had been a single birth, "the [annual health-care] savings would have been more than $3 million in this one hospital."[3]

High Costs at Home

After leaving the hospital, baby-related expenses for multiples can be extremely high. It's estimated that each month, quintuplets need 900 diapers, 200 jars of baby

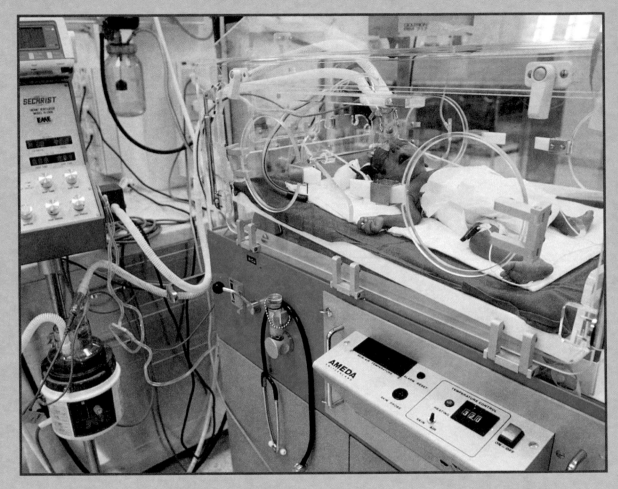

Life-support equipment surrounds an incubator holding a premature infant. Unfortunately, many multiples are born prematurely.

food, 40 gallons of milk, 155 cans of baby formula, and 75 bottles of juice. While these and other related expenses may strain even a comfortable family's income, they can demolish a more modest family budget.

Often, parents of multiples are assisted by government funding, gifts from baby-product manufacturers, and help from family and friends. For the Aymonds, meeting the needs of five new babies on Kirk's salary as a lab technician certainly seemed challenging. Luckily, a local department store volunteered to provide the Aymonds with $250 each month for baby clothing. By waiting for sales and choosing wisely, Denise was able to buy enough to clothe the children for several years. Their transportation problems were solved for a while when a car dealership lent them a van for a year. Their low income also qualified them for a government food program that provided the babies with most of their formula, juice, and cereal. "Without that, we'd be in trouble," Denise noted in reviewing their expenses.[4]

Other families have coped in similar ways with the financial problems brought on by multiple birth. A New York couple attempting to raise quintuplets in a small living space were given a larger apartment by an anonymous benefactor. The Gerber Products Company, which manufactures numerous items for infants and toddlers, even developed the Gerber Multiple Births Program. Designed to ease the financial burden of having triplets, quadruplets, quintuplets, or more, the company provides the parents of these newborns with an array of practical gifts, including baby food and clothing.

Although the costs can be staggering and the workload daunting, most parents of multiples are thrilled to

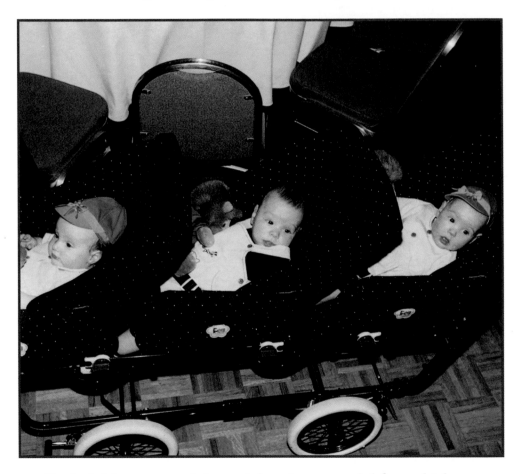

Food, clothing, toys, and the special equipment needed for multiples can become quite expensive.

have their newborns. Often, these instantly large families are the end result of trying a host of fertility treatments after years of failing to have children naturally. As one father described the joy involved, "The best part is that they love us so much. When they see us, their faces light up. That must be a great feeling for a parent with one child, but we have it four times."[5]

Difficult Decisions

Yet for others, the possibility of a multiple birth resulting from fertility treatments is less joyous. These couples find the thought of caring for newborns with severe health problems or handicaps especially sobering. There can be other problems as well. Many multiple pregnancies are never carried to term. In such instances, all the fetuses are miscarried. In response to these concerns, some couples have resorted to a controversial procedure known as **selective reduction.**

During this process, a doctor terminates some of the fetuses in the woman's uterus while leaving the others intact. With selective reduction, the precise position of the fetuses is first detected with an ultrasound scanner. Then a needle filled with potassium chloride is injected into the hearts of the targeted fetuses to stop the fetal heartbeat. The dead fetuses shrivel up and are expelled during the regular delivery or are absorbed by the body during pregnancy. Selective reduction, which is employed

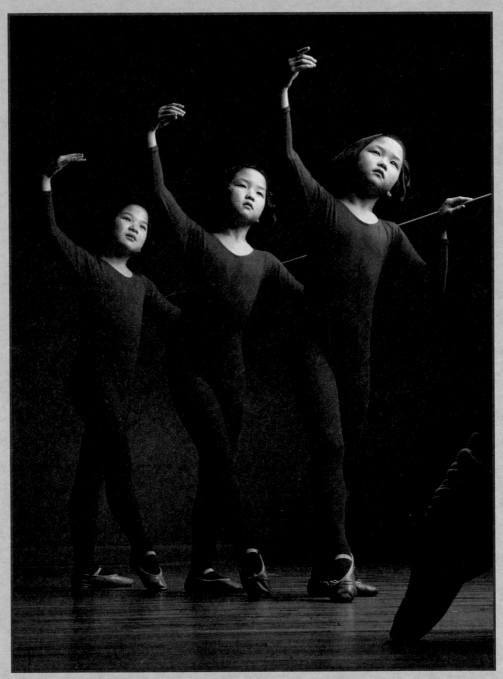

Expenses for multiples continue to grow as the children do. It's dancing lessons today—and college tuition in a few years.

during the first three months of pregnancy, provides both the surviving fetuses and the mother with a better chance for a normal pregnancy and a healthy future.

In a study of the procedure at Mount Sinai School of Medicine in New York City, 85 women each carrying between three and nine fetuses underwent selective reduction with largely favorable results. The remaining fetuses fared well with no infant deaths during delivery or during the often risky first week following birth. There were also no negative physical effects among the mothers as well as less strain on the overall health of these women.

Ethical Issues

Although selective reduction offers women with multiple pregnancies an alternative, it poses a serious ethical issue. Can sacrificing some fetuses to promote the possible well-being of others be morally justified? Kirk and Denise Aymond had refused to even consider the procedure after learning that they were having quintuplets. Determined not to eliminate any of their children, they viewed the babies' chances as either "all of them surviving or none of them surviving."[6]

In the majority of cases where selective reduction is used, the woman is carrying four or more fetuses. In such instances, most doctors would agree that overcrowding the uterus in that manner can result in some babies dying shortly after birth and others being left with permanent disabilities. However, selective reduction becomes especially controversial with women having triplets. At times, such women may choose selective reduction to have twins or even a single child. But with just three fetuses, medical opinions differ as to whether there is any genuinely serious risk to either the fetus or mother. As Susan M. Wolf, a medical **ethicist** from the Hastings Center in Briarcliff Manor, New York, put it, "You are off in the realm of parental preference."[7]

Supporters of selective reduction note that women in the United States can legally terminate a pregnancy during the **first trimester** for any reason at all. They also stress that when choosing selective reduction, parents have no information about the child's gender or other characteristics. This means that no parent can opt for the procedure merely to "choose" the baby's gender or eye color.

But those who are against the procedure claim that while selective reduction is supposedly used only to safeguard the health of the mother and child, it's impossible to know when other factors have actually come into play. Some argue that selective reduction is often chosen by couples who wanted only one child at a time but underwent infertility treatments that gave them more than they bargained for. And some argue that it is the fertility doctors—not the couples—who are to blame for this.

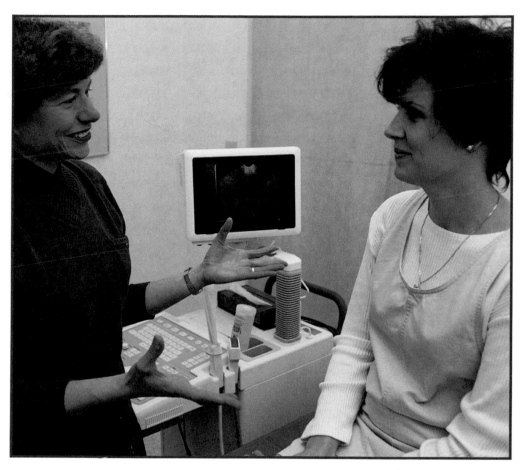

Doctors sometimes discuss the option of selective reduction with patients who are having multiples.

Other moral as well as practical concerns surround the issue of multiple births. Medical-payment records reveal that the high costs associated with multiple births are often at least partially paid for by government funding or health insurance. This means that the general public helps to pay for these consequences through their tax dollars or higher insurance premiums. With health-care funds being so tight, some wonder if infertility treatments, which are largely responsible for the dramatic increase in multiples, should be made readily available to everyone. Moreover, some infertility treatments are more likely to result in multiple births than others. Should physicians center their energy on those most likely to produce a single birth? Firm answers to these highly debatable issues have yet to be determined.

CHAPTER 4

BEING A MULTIPLE

*O*ften, parents of multiples have spoken out on what it's like to have more than one baby at a time. Less is known, however, about what it's like to actually *be* a multiple. Although quintuplets and quadruplets have become increasingly common in recent years, these large families can still attract a great deal of attention in public places.

When a set of New Jersey quintuplets were spotted at a mall recently, a crowd of more than 50 people immediately surrounded the children. Some of the "quint watchers" asked to be photographed with the youngsters.

In the Spotlight

Being born as part of a large group of multiples can mean having your picture in the paper—or perhaps even finding work in television commercials or magazine ads. The 1963 birth of the Harkins quadruplets—Mary, Alice, Beth, and Anita—caused quite a stir in their hometown of Jackson, Mississippi. The mayor proclaimed a special day in the babies' honor and a local clothing store promised to provide the quadruplets with new wardrobes each year. Offers for college scholarships rolled in when the girls were just days old.

All this attention can sometimes be confusing to a young person. Multiples soon realize that they aren't like their friends and classmates. As a result, they may often be wary of their seemingly unfounded popularity. Amy Kienast, one of a set of quintuplets, recalled wondering as a child, "What did we do to become famous? All we did was be born."[1]

Myths Surrounding Multiples

Nevertheless, throughout history, rare qualities have sometimes been attributed to multiples. Among a number of tribes in upper New Guinea, it was believed that a twin could stop a pot of water from boiling just by looking at it. In various early cultures, the birth of multiples might be considered cause for either joyous celebration or human sacrifice. While more research has been focused on twins than on larger groups of multiples, there is enough available evidence to cast doubt on some of the myths surrounding multiples.

Perhaps the most commonly held myth is that all multiples enjoy a close and enduring bond to one another. Although popular culture supports the notion of multiples relating to one another as though they were lifelong best friends, this isn't always the case. Just as relationships vary among other brothers and sisters, so do those of multiples.

A study conducted at the University of Louisville in Kentucky revealed that the bond between twins is not unlike that of any two siblings close in age. Ricardo Ainslie, another researcher working with twins, confirmed these findings. He noted that "twins are not fundamentally different from nontwins." He added that "nontwins raised under similar circumstances, for example siblings who are very close in age, may closely resemble twins psychologically."[2]

In addition, factors such as environment, upbringing, and education can have a bearing on how these relationships develop or change. Some multiples may become

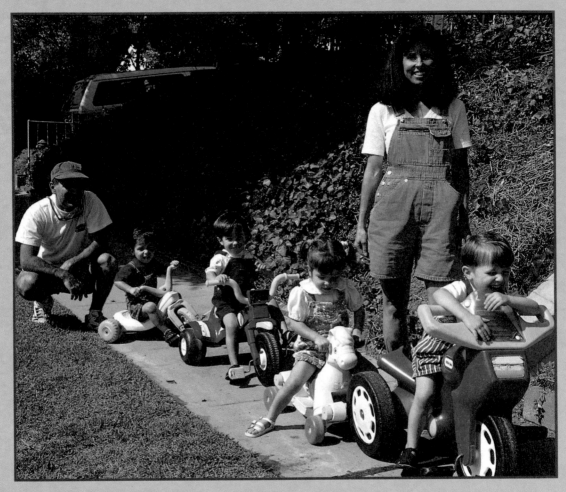

Even though multiples are more common today, cute quadruplets like these can still draw a lot of attention.

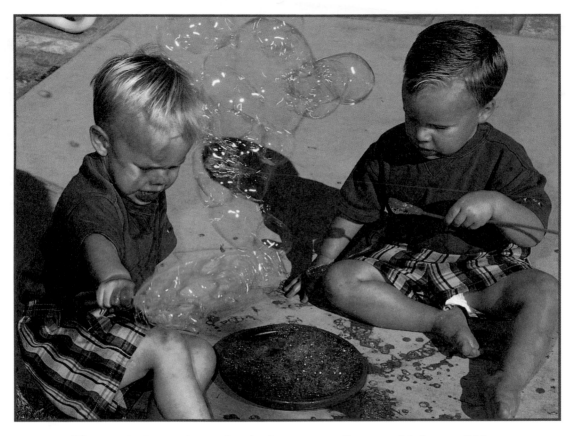

These twin boys enjoy each other's company. Some multiples are lifelong best friends, but this isn't always so.

closer through the years, while others become more distant or competitive. Change may be especially evident during adolescence, when many multiples—just like other teens—begin to focus more on their individuality than on their sibling bonds.

Another myth about multiples is that most multiples can communicate with one another through **ESP (extrasensory perception)** in times of crisis or emergency. Although there are reported cases of ESP among multiples, similar accounts have come from close siblings, husbands and wives, and even good friends. However, many reports of ESP are questionable. Often these incidents have been found to be due to genetics or learned behaviors rather than to supernatural circumstances.

Sympathetic pain—such as a twin feeling pain when the other twin has had surgery—has been rationally explained as well. Some psychologists believe that this happens because twins or other multiples have been together since before birth and know each other so well that they have come to feel for one another on many levels. This explanation sometimes also holds true for married people who are very close—such as when a husband experiences labor pains as his wife is giving birth.

Unique Experiences

Nevertheless, being a multiple does create some unique opportunities for fun. At times, identical twins or triplets have fooled friends, teachers, and dates by pretending to be one another. But there are drawbacks as well. Even when multiples are urged to develop their individuality, they are usually first seen by others—especially in their early years—as "one of" the quintuplets, quadruplets, etc.

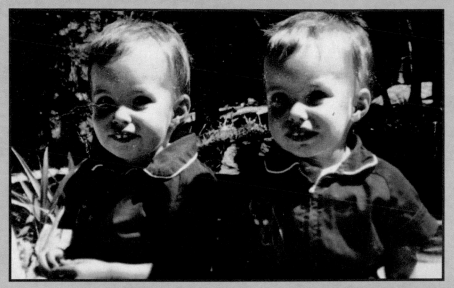

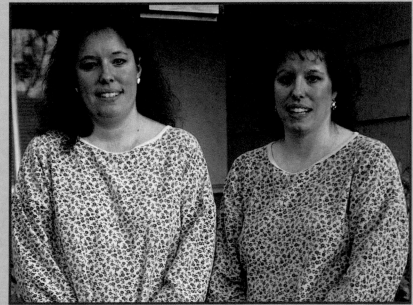

Identical multiples often look very much alike when they are young, but less so when they are older. At 18 months of age, it's hard to tell these twin sisters apart, but at 35 years of age, you can easily tell one sister from the other.

This invites comparisons, and at times these distinctions can be painful. For example all four of the Harkins quadruplets were good students, but one term, Mary failed to make the honor roll while the other three did. When the names of those on the honor roll were announced, she overheard a classmate say, "Mary must be the dumb one."[3]

While all multiples grow and develop in their own way, the Harkins quadruplets, now adults, have always remained close. In describing their tightly knit bond, one sister noted that remaining in tune with one another was "just a way of life for us."[4] As further research is done on multiples, we may learn more about what it's like to grow up as one. Yet some people insist that it's impossible to ever thoroughly define or classify certain types of very personal relationships. As one of the Harkins quadruplets noted, "You'd have . . . to be born . . . together . . . to understand."[5]

GLOSSARY

CEREBRAL PALSY a disability resulting from damage to the brain before, during, or shortly after birth; it causes muscular and speech problems

CESAREAN SECTION a surgical procedure, used when a normal birth is dangerous or not possible, in which an infant is delivered through an incision made in the mother's abdomen and uterus

EGG the female reproductive cell

ENDORSEMENT an agreement to support or stand behind a product or person

EXTRASENSORY PERCEPTION (ESP) to have knowledge about a person, place, or incident without using the five known senses (sight, taste, hearing, smell, or touch)

ETHICIST a person who studies human conduct with an emphasis on the determination of right and wrong

FETUS the developing infant in its mother's uterus

FIRST TRIMESTER the first three months of pregnancy

HORMONAL caused by hormones; hormones are bodily secretions released into the bloodstream in tiny amounts by a specific gland or tissue

INFERTILITY the inability of a man or woman to produce a child because of physical problems

INTENSIVE CARE   medical equipment and services provided for seriously ill patients

IN VITRO FERTILIZATION   a process through which eggs are taken from a woman's body, fertilized by sperm in a lab, and then reinserted into her body

MIDWIFE   a woman who assists in delivering babies

MISCARRY   to lose a fetus before it has developed enough to survive outside the uterus

OVARIES   the two reproductive organs in women that produce eggs and female sex hormones

PREMATURE   a baby born too early—having been in its mother's uterus less than nine months

PROFITEERING   seeking to gain excessive profits at someone else's expense

RESPIRATORY THERAPIST   a medical technician who monitors and takes care of breathing difficulties in premature babies caused by underdeveloped lungs

SELECTIVE REDUCTION   a procedure in which a doctor removes some fetuses by injection to improve the survival chances of the remaining fetuses in the womb

UTERUS   the organ of female mammals in which the young develop before birth; also called the womb

SOURCE NOTES

CHAPTER ONE
1. Barry Came, "A Family Tragedy," *Maclean's*, November 21, 1994, 41.

2. Ibid.

3. Ibid.

4. Ibid., 42.

5. Tom Fennell, "The Forgotten Dionnes," *Maclean's*, November 21, 1994, 45.

6. Barry Came, 43.

7. Ibid.

8. Fennell, 44.

CHAPTER TWO
1. Dianne Hales, "The Baby-Baby-Baby Boom!!!" *Redbook*, January 1989, 96.

2. "The High Cost of Having Some Babies . . . Gets Higher by the Numbers," *Science News*, August 6, 1994, 95.

3. Dianne Hales, 97.

CHAPTER THREE
1. Martha Raddatz, "Raising Quints," *Parents*, October 1994, 19.

2. Ibid.

3. "The High Cost of Having Some Babies . . .Gets Higher by the Numbers," 95.

4. Martha Raddatz, 22.

5. Ingrid Groller, "And Baby Makes Six," *Parents*, November 1988, 134.

6. Martha Raddatz, 18.

7. R. A. Fackelmann, "Experimental Method Lowers Multifetal Risk," *Science News*, May 5, 1990, 279.

CHAPTER FOUR
1. Steve Dougherty, "A Not So Singular Sensation at Birth: The Kienast Quints Turn 21 and Take a Fond Look Back," *People*, March 11, 1991, 118.

2. Pamela Patrick Novotny, *The Joy of Twins; Having, Raising and Loving Babies Who Arrive in Groups* (New York: Crown Publishers, 1988), 248.

3. Dennis Covington, "The Mysterious World of Quadruplets," *Redbook*, April 1996, 107.

4. Ibid., 106.

5. Ibid., 134.

ORGANIZATIONS & PUBLICATIONS

BOOKS

Anderson, Joan. **Twins on Toes: A Ballet Debut.** New York: Lodestar, 1993.

Cohen, Shari. **Coping with Sibling Rivalry.** New York: Rosen Publications, 1989.

Feldman, Robert S. **Who Are You? Personality and Its Development.** Danbury, CT: Franklin Watts, 1992.

Jenness, Aylette. **Families: A Celebration of Diversity, Commitment, and Love.** Boston: Houghton Mifflin, 1989.

Landau, Elaine. **Sibling Rivalry.** Brookfield, CT: Millbrook Press, 1994.

LeShan, Eda J. **What Makes You So Special?** New York: Dial Books For Young Readers, 1992.

Livingston, Cohn Myra. **Poems for Brothers, Poems for Sisters.** New York: Holiday House, 1991.

Rosenberg, Maxine. **Being a Twin; Having a Twin.** New York: Lothrop, Lee & Shepard, 1985.

Rosenberg, Maxine. **Finding a Way: Living with Exceptional Brothers and Sisters.** New York: Lothrop, Lee, & Shepard.

ORGANIZATIONS
The Center for the Study of Multiple Births
333 East Superior Street, Suite 463-5
Chicago, IL 60601

International Twins Association, Inc.
6898 Channel Road
Minneapolis, MN 55432

The International Twins Foundation
P.O. Box 6043
Providence, RI 02940
e-mail: *TwinsFdn@aol.com*

Triplet Connection
P.O Box 99571
Stockton, CA 95209
e-mail: *Triplets@inreach.com*

Twins and Multiple Births Association (TAMBA)
P.O. Box 30
Little Sutton
South Wirral, L66 1TH
England
Great Britain

Twins Day Festival Committee
P.O. Box 29
Twinsburg, OH 44087

RESOURCES ON THE WORLD WIDE WEB

NATIONAL ORGANIZATION OF MOTHERS OF TWINS CLUBS
http://www. parentsplace.com/readroom/momsoftwins/

PARENTS OF TWINS/MULTIPLES
Discussion areas, resources, links, and frequently asked questions.
http://www.Ind.com/twins

THE TRIPLET CONNECTION
All kinds of information about twins, triplets, and multiple births, including news, services, Q&A, directories, stories, and links.
http://www.inreach.com/triplets/

TWINS MAGAZINE
Constantly changing online magazine featuring articles on the multiple-birth family.
http://www. twinsmagazine.com/

TwinSource

The science and study of twins and famous twins in history, plus links to support networks, stories, the Twins Day Festival, and lots more.

http://www.modcult.brown.edu/students/angell/ TWINSource.html

Twins Support Groups and Services

Dozens of links to organizations related to twins and multiple births, including support groups and services.

http://www. visi.com/~johnr/twinrefs.html

INDEX

Page numbers in *italics* indicate illustrations.

ABOUT THE
AUTHOR

ELAINE LANDAU has a Bachelor of Arts degree in English and Journalism from New York University and a Master's degree in Library and Information Science from Pratt Institute. She has worked as a newspaper reporter, children's book editor, and a youth services librarian, but especially enjoys writing for young people.

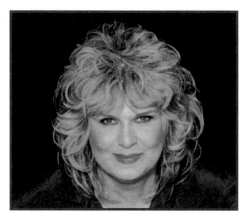

Ms. Landau has written more than 100 nonfiction books on various topics. She lives in Miami, Florida, with her husband, Norman, and son, Michael.